Gaining Freedom from Sex Addictions:

Breaking Free of Pornography and Prostitutes

Matthew Robert Payne

To sow into Matthew's writing ministry, to request a personal prophecy or life-coaching session, or to contact him, please visit http://personal-prophecy-today.com

Cover designed by akira007 at fiverr.com.

Edited by Lisa Thompson at www.writebylisa.com You can email Lisa at writebylisa@gmail.com

Published by Revival Waves of Glory Books & Publishing PO Box 596| Litchfield, Illinois 62056 USA

Revival Waves of Glory Books & Publishing is committed to excellence in the publishing industry. Their website is www.revivalwavesofgloryministries.com

Paperback: 978-1-68411-403-0

Hardcover: 978-1-68411-404-7

Dedication

I want to dedicate this book to the Holy Spirit who leads me, encourages me, and helps me in all that I do. He is an unknown and unrecognized hero in Christian circles. He puts himself last and doesn't promote himself but gives me the power to overcome sin and do all that I do.

He is the power source in this verse.

Ephesians 3:20 - Now to Him who is able to do exceedingly abundantly above all that we ask or think, according to the power that works in us.

Acknowledgements

Father God

I want to thank you for loving me, for leading me, and for making me into the person that I am today. I thank you for loving me through all the years of my addictions. Thank you for your Son, my best friend. Thank you for your Holy Spirit.

Jesus Christ

Thank you for being my friend for all of my life. I cannot thank you enough for all that you do for me. I live to serve you and do everything that you call me to do. I cannot imagine life without you. Thank you for loving me through all the years until I was set free. I thank you and the Holy Spirit each day for guiding me.

Bill Vincent

I want to thank Bill Vincent, who produces my paperback books, my e-books, and my audio books. His company, Revival Waves of Glory Books & Publishing, has shown me great favor, and without you, I would be spending a lot more money to produce books. I give you my heartfelt thanks.

Lisa Thompson

I want to thank my editor who works really hard on all the books that I currently produce. If you need editing or proofreading for your book, contact Lisa at www.writebylisa.com or by email at writebylisa@gmail.com

The Readers

I want to thank my readers. I hope that you enjoy this book, and I am praying for you to find the courage and the path to freedom.

Ministry Supporters

I want to thank all the people who have requested a prophecy from me, people who have requested a life-coaching session, or your own message from an angel. I want to thank all those who have sown into my book-writing ministry. Without you, this book would not have been possible.

June and Bob Payne

I want to thank my mother and father for all of their love and support of me.

A Note from My Editor

Wow. I have just finished the first round of edits for *Gaining Freedom from Sex Addictions: Breaking Free of Pornography and Prostitutes*, and I am very impressed! Matthew handles an extremely difficult subject with grace and tact, yet he confronts the issues that men and women face head on.

With his typical style of candor and honesty, Matthew relays how he gained freedom from addictions of thirty-six years to pornography and twenty-five years to prostitutes. His message of hope for all reverberates throughout the pages of this book.

This book does not offer easy solutions or a specific "formula." Instead, Matthew provides the reader with step-by-step actions to take in order to secure freedom. The most foundational and strategic of these is reframing your mindset and understanding your identity in Christ. Once you see yourself as Christ sees you, you will then be able to move forward into the freedom Christ has for you.

I believe that this powerful manuscript will bring freedom to many. If you or a loved one has struggled with sexual addictions, be encouraged! I am declaring hope to you as you read these pages, and I am believing that you will find true and lasting victory in Jesus.

Please feel free to contact me at www.writebylisa.com or at my direct e-mail at writebylisa@gmail.com if you have any questions about editing.

Blessings,

Lisa

Table of Contents

Dedication.......... iii

Acknowledgements iv

A Note from My Editor vi

Chapter 1 - My History 1

Chapter 2 - You Are not Alone.......... 7

Chapter 3 - This Problem Is a Real Problem 15

Chapter 4 - God Loves You in the Midst of Your Struggles 19

Chapter 5 - Striving Won't Fix It 24

Chapter 6 - You Are Perfect.......... 30

Chapter 7 - You Are Holy and Blameless 38

Chapter 8 - You Are Inhabitants of a Brand New Kingdom 44

Chapter 9 - You Are Righteous, Peaceful, and Joyful 47

Chapter 10 - Coming to True Repentance.......... 53

Chapter 11 - God's Grace Is the Answer 58

Chapter 12 - Walking out Your Freedom.......... 63

I'd love to hear from you.......... 68

How to Sponsor a Book Project.......... 70

Other Books by Matthew Robert Payne 71

About Matthew Robert Payne 74

Chapter 1 – My History

Ephesians 2:8-10 - For by grace you have been saved through faith, and that not of yourselves; *it is* the gift of God, not of works, lest anyone should boast. For we are His workmanship, created in Christ Jesus for good works, which God prepared beforehand that we should walk in them.

Ephesians 3:20 - Now to Him who is able to do exceedingly abundantly above all that we ask or think, according to the power that works in us.

Romans 8:28 - And we know that all things work together for good to those who love God, to those who are the called according to *His* purpose.

Unfortunately, when I was growing up, my father had with an angry disposition, and I was somewhat afraid of him. My older brother dealt with a little bit of sibling rivalry, and he used to hit me and pick on me. My mother told me that she couldn't leave him alone in a room with me because he was so violent toward me.

I had a temperamental and sad start to life. At eight years of age, my cat died. I had mourned the cat for six months when a child evangelist came to my town. The evangelist said that we could have a friend named Jesus who would never leave us or forsake us. Since I really missed my cat that was my friend and I lost him, I accepted Jesus into my life. From that day on, I was saved, like the above verse says. "For by grace you have been saved through faith, and that not of yourselves; it is the gift of God."

Getting free of pornography or prostitution is done by faith and is a gift of God. You can't do it by works; you can't do it by striving. At eight years of age, I was saved. At fourteen years of age, I was molested on the beach by a homosexual/pedophile. I then began a life of having sexual encounters with men on a nudist beach.

At the age of fourteen, I had my first orgasm. I then learned to be aroused by naked women on a nudist beach. I started to buy pornography and became addicted to it at this age. At the same time, I struggled with singing in church, and I couldn't praise Jesus because I was feeling so guilty for my involvement with porn and for being with men on the beach whenever I went to surf.

At the age of eighteen, I moved away from my town in the country and into the city. I slept with a street-walking prostitute who took me to her room upstairs. I soon learned that you could hire more expensive prostitutes and hire expensive women called "escorts." You could call their agency and have them come to your house. Seeing escorts costs a lot of money, and I stayed perpetually broke. For twenty-five years while I was addicted to prostitutes, I never bought a house and had little financial stability. Proverbs 29:3b says, ". . . a companion of prostitutes squanders his wealth" (ESV). Satan really steals from you however he can.

In the midst of my sinful life, God has still been able to use me to prophesy 20,000 times and to write twenty-eight books. This is despite the fact that I failed English in high school. Ephesians 3:20 says, "Now to Him who is able to do exceedingly abundantly above all that we ask or think, according to the power that works in us."

God has used someone who failed English to write twenty-eight books to minister to thousands of people. This month as I currently produce this book, 1,800 people have downloaded one of my books for 99 cents.

I had a twenty-five-year addiction to prostitutes from the ages of eighteen to forty-three before I was set free about eight years ago. In the midst of those addictions, God still used me.

Romans 8:28 says, "And we know that all things work together for good, for those who love God, and are called according to his purpose." That purpose is the good things that God prepared beforehand that we should walk in them mentioned in Ephesians 2:10. Now I'm a writer, a prophet, and a minister of the Gospel. I'm touching lives; I'm saving lives, and I am now free from my addiction to pornography and prostitutes.

We will talk about being set free from pornography and from an addiction to prostitutes. Many people who are addicted to prostitutes have a history of addiction to porn as well. Pornography increases the prostitution addiction as people are used to seeing girls in porn and want to act out what they have seen.

I am writing a book to give people hope and to share how I gained my freedom. Perhaps this book won't have all the answers for you, and perhaps you will also need counseling for inner healing and personal deliverance. You might even need to join a program that works with people addicted to pornography. Whatever you choose, this book is mainly centered and targeted toward people who have or who have had an addiction to pornography or who currently visit prostitutes or who have done so in the past. I am offering a message of hope to say, "I've been there. I've lived it. I've been set free. I've come out of it, and you can, too."

The quoted verse continues, "For we are his workmanship created in Christ Jesus for good works, which God has prepared beforehand that we should walk in them." In the last six months, I've been set free from pornography.

I pray that you enjoy reading this book, that you are encouraged, and that you can gain something from it. Hopefully, you will be able to speak about this topic with some of your close friends. I know this subject is a very private matter, but part of getting free is confessing this sin and bringing it out into the open with people that you respect and trust.

That's the brief overview of my history with prostitutes and pornography. I will share more throughout the book.

Chapter 2 – You Are not Alone

I searched for some statistics that I will reference here. You can read those statistics for yourself, and I hope that this information comforts you so that you know that you are not alone.

One of the lies of the enemy is that no one else is doing this. When you are visiting prostitutes when you are paid every two weeks or once a month, you suffer alone. You can’t open up about this subject to your friends at church. You can’t say, "Hey, I always sleep with prostitutes, and I am a real loser. I can’t attract a woman who will love me, and I can't have a girlfriend or a wife. I have a strong sex drive, and I just can't help myself. I find that I have to sleep with prostitutes."

You might be married, but your wife is not responding to you sexually. Perhaps she's had children, and she doesn’t want to have sex anymore. Maybe your relationship has become cold. Your wife might not perform for you in the bedroom the way that you've seen in pornography or that you've heard in men’s magazines. Perhaps your wife doesn’t perform sexually to the level that your lust or cravings desire, so you have now decided to fulfill that desire with prostitutes.

The statistics indicate that 15.7 percent of men in Australia have visited a prostitute once in their lifetime, and 15 to 20 percent of men in America have visited a prostitute. Men visit prostitutes for many reasons. Maybe you have been rejected or received wounds in your life that cause you to seek, to watch, or to look at pornography on the internet. Perhaps you practice your habit when your wife is out or when she is not around. If you're a single male, perhaps every time you turn on your computer, you find yourself visiting a pornography site.

Personally, I was simply bored with life. I reached a point when I was not doing anything. Pornography used to excite me and give me something to do and look at. I had my favorite forms of porn in a certain video, in certain sexual scenes that I won't describe. I searched for that specific type of pornography, and I used to watch that. I just couldn't help myself.

The lie of Satan is that you're the only one viewing porn, but the statistics say that 3 out of every 10 Christian men between the ages of eighteen and thirty view pornography daily.[1] This means that if three men are sitting together in church, one of you is watching porn every day. In a church of a hundred people with fifty men, fifteen of them are watching pornography every day. You are not alone.

An estimated 3 percent of Christian women in the same age group also reportedly access porn every day. Satan lies to you and keeps you bound.

When you live with the shame and the condemnation of pornography, then you can be seriously hurt and negatively affected by it if you are watching it every day. You might never get to the place where you feel good about yourself. You are always suffering in condemnation and in guilt. You are always feeling guilty and as if God doesn't love you. You don't feel acceptable or think that you measure up, and you think that you are a failure. Satan tells you, "What kind of Christian are you that you are always masturbating and always looking at porn?"

---

[1] Pelletier, Joseph. 2016. "NEW SURVEY OF PORN USE: MEN AND WOMEN WATCHING IN STARTLING NUMBERS." Church Militant. https://www.churchmilitant.com/news/article/new-survey-of-porn-use-shows-startling-stats-for-men-and-women.

If you are seeing prostitutes, you feel like you're a loser. You deal with a lot of guilt and shame after the act and suffer the financial lack as well, the gap in your wallet. When you go and see a prostitute, it costs money, money that you can't really afford.

A lot of pornography is free, so it's not costing men a lot of money. Satan wants you to live in shame, but Romans 8:1 says "There is now no condemnation to those who are in Christ Jesus, who do not walk according to the flesh but according to the spirit."

Jesus wants you to know that you're loved and that condemnation for your sin doesn't come from him. Condemnation doesn't come from Jesus Christ, and he loves you. The enemy wants to keep porn a secret in your life. You might be open and share that you have a pornography problem. However, if you're sharing this with other people who also have a porn problem, they really don't have the answers for you. If you're sharing with the pastor who's never had a pornography problem, he might not have the answers for you and might not be able understand you or help you with your journey. If you're sleeping with prostitutes, you have to be very open about what's going on to actually admit that you’re sleeping with prostitutes.

Satan wants you to think that you're the only one, that you can't confess your sin, that you can't share this with people. Yet part of the journey to freedom is to be open and honest and to be able to share what you're going through.

Please read over the following statistics.

Pornography

Charisma magazine reported the following: “A national survey of Christian men reveals shocking statistics pertaining to high rates of pornography use and addiction and rampant sexual infidelity among married Christian men.

“The 2014 survey was commissioned by a nonprofit organization called Proven Men Ministries and conducted by Barna Group among a nationally representative sample of 388 self-identified Christian adult men.

“Those who identify themselves as born-again Christians have similar struggles with pornography and affairs:

- 95 percent admit that they have viewed pornography.
- 54 percent look at pornography at least once a month.
- 44 percent viewed pornography at work in the last ninety days.
- 31 percent had a sexual affair while married.
- 25 percent erase internet browsing history to conceal pornography use.
- 18 percent admit being addicted to pornography (and another 9 percent think they may be).[2]

The same study further claims three out of every ten men between the ages of eighteen and thirty view porn daily; 3 percent of women in the same age group purportedly access pornography daily.[3]

My deliverance counselor at Freedom Encounters said that at least 90 percent of the men who come in for deliverance have a pornography

---

[2] Staff. 2014. "Shocker: Study Shows Most Christian Men Are Into Porn." *Charisma.* http://www.charismanews.com/us/45671-shocker-study-shows-most-christian-men-are-into-porn.

[3] Pelletier, Joseph. 2016. "NEW SURVEY OF PORN USE: MEN AND WOMEN WATCHING IN STARTLING NUMBERS." *Church Militant.* https://www.churchmilitant.com/news/article/new-survey-of-porn-use-shows-startling-stats-for-men-and-women.

issue. If you feel that you need ministry in this area, contact Freedom Encounters for help.

Prostitutes

The online magazine, *50-ish.org,* related the following information. "Procon.org compiled global studies between 1994 and 2010 and then presented their findings in The Johns Chart.

"On the low side, 15 percent of men have used the services of a prostitute at least once in the USA and 20 percent on the high side.

"15.7 percent of men in Australia have visited a prostitute at least once.

"Men who pay for sex are often portrayed as middle-aged, successful, professional individuals that work long hours and travel away from home quite a bit. But in reality, studies have revealed that there are no obvious stereotypical types that partake in pay for play.

"What research can conclude is that the bulk of promiscuous men are between eighteen and seventy years of age. Those with religious convictions or those who work in 'moral' occupations are not spared from the lure of secretive sex with streetwalkers, call girls, or brothel workers. The powerful and natural sex instinct can, and does, deliver all kinds of men into the arms of sex workers.

"The majority of men that sleep with prostitutes share the following:

- They're educated beyond the high school level
- In regular, full-time employment.
- Respected members of society
- Seem to be decent people
- Display good manners and social skills.
- At least 50 percent are married or in long-term relationships."[4]

[4] Strowger, Toby. 2014. "Why do Men Sleep with Prostitutes?" *50-ish.org.* http://www.50ish.org/lifestyle/why-do-men-sleep-with-prostitutes/

Chapter 3 – This Problem Is a Real Problem

This problem is a real problem that you cannot fix on your own. We are called the Body of Christ for a specific reason; we are meant to be a body that functions together. Men and women are meant to have others of the same gender that they can confide in and be honest with.

When a married man is viewing pornography regularly, this can seriously affect his wife. Some men start to become sexual deviants in the bedroom and ask the wife to perform sexual duties and acts that she is not happy with.

The fact that the man is looking at stunning women who are porn stars can make the women feel unloved, unappreciated, unattractive, plain, and ugly to her husband. When a woman realizes that her husband is not having sex with her but is watching porn and using it to satisfy himself, then the problem is bigger than just a man with a porn addiction.

It's also a problem for the wife. She also has to go through healing for the wounds that this causes. The man needs to have men who he can talk to, such as a pastor or other people that can empathize with him and understand him. He needs people to listen to him, not condemn or judge him but to bring correction, support, and encouragement to him so that he can do his best to heal.

I shared Ephesians 2:8-9 earlier. “For by grace you’ve been saved through faith. It’s not of yourselves, it’s a gift of God. Not of works that anyone should boast.” God must act to free you from pornography. You will need his help in your life so that the temptations actually stop. I found that, for me, getting free of pornography was a process, and, when I reached a certain stage, the temptation to engage in pornography actually stopped.

Up until that point in my life, the temptation came in as a ten out of ten. When the temptations stopped, the temptation came in at just one out of ten, and I could easily dismiss and disregard it. I've been so happy since being free of it.

You need the help of God. You need the understanding, the prayer, and the support of other men. If you're a woman who’s struggling with pornography, I'd suggest you see other women and go through the same process that I'm talking about in this book. As a man, I am obviously addressing men.

You have to understand that if you have an addiction to pornography or to seeing prostitutes, you have a real problem. You cannot minimize it. It will take away your energy and your spirit. It will lead you into guilt, condemnation, and shame. It will take away your peace and joy. In some instances, it might take the presence of God from your life. You can cause yourself and your family financial problems and strain. Satan will just rob and steal from you and ultimately, destroy you.

You need to come to a place where you're honest with yourself and where you admit that you're addicted. If you are watching a pornography website daily, weekly, or monthly, you have a problem. Of course, the more often you see porn, the bigger the problem is, but sin is still sin, and even if you view it once a month, you will be plagued with guilt, shame, and condemnation. When you have a porn addiction or an addiction to prostitutes, you have a real problem.

I am sure some men who are not Christians can overcome a pornography addiction or an addiction to prostitutes. I personally needed the grace of God and the power that's found in that grace to set me free from the addiction to prostitutes.

I am very happy in the place where I am now. I love going to church because I no longer need to start worship by confessing my sins. I no longer have to come before God to repent of my pornography addiction so that I can be in the right place and free from the guilt, shame, and condemnation of the enemy so that I can worship God. I am so relieved to walk into a church without any sin on my mind and without any consciousness of sin that I've committed in the last few days. I had to come to grips with the fact that this was a real problem and that I needed God to help me.

Chapter 4 – God Loves You in the Midst of Your Struggles

One of the most important lessons that you can learn from this book or from any theology or any other teaching is that God loves you regardless of your sin. You have to come to a place where you understand that you are a son of God, and you are adopted into the family of God through the blood of Jesus Christ, and you're holy and righteous before him. You need to come to a place where you understand that before you sin, while you sin, and after you sin, God still loves you just the same. Stop and think about that for a minute.

God doesn't leave you when you're about to see a prostitute and only return after you've confessed. God doesn't leave you as you log on to an internet site when you are going to watch pornography. God doesn't leave and turn his head away from you. He is still there, and he is still watching, and he still loves you. He doesn't turn his love off and on, depending on if you repent and confess and return to him.

When you opened the internet site and watched the porn or when you gave yourself to the prostitute, you move away from him. You start to move away from him, from his direction, his Spirit, and his presence. You are the one who actively pursues the sin and practices it. You have moved away from God.

The situation is similar to a little boy who has done something really bad that his father told him not to do. The father knows that something is wrong because the boy is not acting as loving as usual, and he is being distant toward him. The father will pick up on the fact that something is wrong and ask the boy, "What's the matter with you?" God is the same way. The son's guilt puts a wedge between him and his father.

God is waiting for your embrace; he is waiting to grab you and hug you and pour out his love on you and show you that he loves you. The prodigal son found himself in a pig pen, feeding pigs. He had spent all of his father's inheritance on prostitutes and wild living and a prodigal lifestyle. That's why this parable is called the "prodigal son." Instead, it should be really called "a loving father." The son came back and wanted to work as a servant, and he had his speech ready, everything that he was going to say and promise his father. He started to confess and say all he planned to say, but his father shut him up and put a robe on him, put some sandals on his feet, gave him a signet ring, and threw a party for him.

The next time that you are in the middle of your sin, think of that story. That's how God feels about you. In the midst of your sin, in the midst of your depravity, in the midst of who you are, you must understand that God's love for you does not change. Let that truth permeate your spirit.

When you're sleeping with prostitutes or falling into the sin of pornography, knowing that you are still loved is one of the most important lessons that you need to learn before you can be set free. Selah.

Joseph Prince in his book, *Destined to Reign*, teaches on this. When you are moving in a cycle of guilt and condemnation, your guilt and your shame will pull you back into the sin to repeat it. We can actually become addicted to feeling worthless and to feeling bad about ourselves.

We actually crave the feeling of feeling bad. Sadly, we go back to participate in the sin again so that we can feel that shame, worthlessness, and unhappiness that tells us that we are not worth anything.

I was having encounters with saints and angels about a year ago. Every time an angel, a saint, or Jesus showed up, I immediately thought of my sin of pornography. Satan instantly lied to me, “You're not worthy to be talking to these angels and holy people because you’re masturbating to porn.”

One day, my scribe angel spoke to me. She showed up, and I thought of the porn. She said, "Matthew, I want to tell you something."

I responded, "What?"

She answered, "Your sin does not define you. The pornography does not define you. You are a beautiful person, and Jesus really loves you. You need to come to grips with the fact that you are loved. Jesus isn't turning his back on you when you sin. I love you for who you are, and you need to accept that Jesus loves you for who you are."

A week later, Bob Jones, a former prophet on earth, visited me from heaven. I was walking down the road with him. When he appeared, I started thinking about the pornography, and he told me, "What Bethany, your angel, told you is true. Your sin doesn’t define you, Matthew. We don’t think of you as such a bad masturbator or such a bad porn addict. We don’t ask how God copes with you.”

He continued, "Like your angel, Bethany, told you, you sin doesn’t define you. This is what you are like. You're honest, transparent, loving, passionate, teachable, humble, dependable, and faithful.” He listed about twenty attributes of what heaven thought of me. My eyes filled with tears.

"When we think of you, that’s what we think of. We think of those twenty things that you are; we don’t think of your sin. You need a little bit more inner healing, and this pornography sin will be gone from your life. This will be Satan’s last stand in your life.”

I was really encouraged by what Bob said that day, reinforcing what Bethany, my angel, had said. A short time later, I went to counseling and received some inner healing so that I was finally free from pornography.

Chapter 5 – Striving Won't Fix It

If you're addicted to prostitutes or to pornography and if you can admit that you're addicted, you have taken the first step in facing your problem. This is the path to healing. Watching porn once a month is a problem. Watching porn once a week is a bigger problem. Watching porn every day is more of an issue, and some people even watch it many times per day.

The established church teaches us, "Don't do this. Don't do that. If you do, you will go to hell." But sadly, many times, the established church doesn't seem to teach people how to be free from these addictions. I want to share some more of my testimony.

For years, I was addicted to prostitutes, and I was going every two weeks when I received my pension payment. When I had a job, I was going weekly and even more often if I could, depending on how much money I had at the time.

Once, I was with a pastor in church, and I swore at him, saying, "Don't tell me that you're going to pray for me. Help me. Show me how to get free of this prostitute addiction."

I went to an inner healing course from Elijah House Ministries. I encourage you to check them out and learn about inner healing and then actually go through the process of inner healing.

I went through this course, which taught on true repentance and what that looks like. It compared how Saul disobeyed Samuel and started a sacrifice when he was told to wait for Samuel. Samuel came, but Saul had already started a sacrifice, and Samuel rebuked him. Saul made an excuse. "The people were pressuring me." He said that he was sorry, but he wasn't really sorry because he was making excuses.

Then, they compared it to when David slept with Bathsheba, and Nathan, the prophet, said, "Imagine a man has a hundred sheep and another man has one sheep, and the man with a hundred sheep takes the sheep of the man who only has one sheep. What would you do?"

David replied, "I'd punish this man."

Nathan announced, "That man is you." David honestly repented of his sin. God still allowed his firstborn son, the baby he conceived with Bathsheba, to die. David washed his face when the child died. He changed his clothes and came out of mourning. He presented himself to God and said, "He cannot come back to me, but someday, I will go to him." David was truly repentant and agreed that he had done wrong. (See 2 Samuel 12.)

After that course at Elijah House Ministries, I went to speak to a counselor, and I shared that I wanted to be free from my prostitution addiction. The counselor listened to me and told me, "Honestly, all I can hear from you is pride, Matthew. You seem to think that you are a good customer to these girls and that you're treating them well."

He continued, "What you're actually doing to these girls is raping them. Many of them have been molested and sexually abused before. They've gone into prostitution because their father or step-father or another man abused them. Every time you pay for sex with them and sleep with them, you're raping them.

“You must come to grips with the fact that you're an abuser, that you're hurting them, and that you're not treating them well. You think that you are helping them by giving them money so that they can earn a living, but you are actually abusing them. Until you can come to grips with the fact that you're sexually abusing them and that you're abusing yourself, abusing the temple of the Lord, things won’t change. You're wasting your money, and you're spending God's precious resources on something that you shouldn’t be spending it on. Until you're sorry for treating them that way and until you're sorry for treating yourself that way, you'll never be free from this.

"You need to honestly do some thinking and gather up all your strength and be truly sorry for abusing women and for abusing yourself and truly sorry for upsetting God. When you reach that point, you can repent, and God will set you free."

I did that the next week at church, and I prayed out loud and said a prayer of repentance, and God set me free.

That worked for prostitution, and I was free. But I tried and tried and tried to be free from porn, and striving just didn’t do it. Trying to stop just didn't work. I needed many wounds healed—wounds of rejection, fear, worry, and feeling unloved by my father. I needed all of those wounds to be healed through prayers and counseling. I needed soul ties broken off between me and the women that I watched in pornography. I needed soul ties broken off my life with my former wife. I needed all sorts of wounds healed, and I also needed deliverance with demonic spirits cast out.

There's a reason behind why you're viewing pornography. There's a reason behind why you seek out the services of prostitutes. You have unhealed emotional wounds in your life. Until those emotional wounds are healed, you might go through deliverance, but the demons will come right back to you because they are attracted to those wounds.

Like me, you might need the process of inner healing, deliverance, and then, you need God's grace. You need to accept that God loves you in the midst of your sin and doesn't love you any less and that you're righteous, holy, and blameless before him even in the midst of your sin. You must come to the understanding of who you are and that you need inner healing and deliverance.

You must throw your whole life into God's hands and say, "I can't do this, God. I'm at the end of myself. Please deliver me." Otherwise, you might not get free.

I got to the point in my life where I went through this process. Then, suddenly, out of nowhere, the temptation stopped, and I was free from pornography. I can't take any credit for it. It was a miracle and still remains a miracle, and I can't teach you how to be free, but I do know the process.

For me, getting freedom was a combination of the right theology, repentance, inner healing, deliverance, and the grace of God. Over the next four chapters, we will look at the right theology. These four chapters are taken from my book, "*Your Identity in Christ*." I highly recommend that you read the whole book.

Chapter 6 – You Are Perfect

The idea that we are already perfect might be foreign to you, but it is still very true. Many people who live in this world are unaware of the salvation that is possible through Christ; even people who are living a Christian life are unaware of that. Through the Holy Spirit dwelling in them, they are already complete and equipped for every good work that God has planned for them.

2 Timothy 3:17 . . . that the man of God may be complete, thoroughly equipped for every good work.

Many people are unaware that they are made up of spirit, soul, and body. When the Holy Spirit comes into a person and starts to reside in our human body, the spirit in us is perfect. From that point on, God sees us as he saw his own Son while he was on earth. Many people might say that the sin they commit each day or week nullifies the assertion that they are perfect. But Scripture says that the son of God and daughter of God have been perfected forever.

Hebrews 10:14 - For by one offering, He has perfected forever those who are being sanctified.

When we are born again and when our spirits are renewed by the infilling of the Holy Spirit, we are made perfect and prepared to do the good deeds that God planned for us to do. The same Holy Spirit that rested on Jesus rests on us. However, our failure to understand these truths stops the will of God in our lives.

Think about it. God's Holy Spirit does not come in half, three-quarters, and full measure. The Holy Spirit comes down to equip us to live out God's will.

I have prayed for about four hundred people to receive the gift of prophecy since I have been a prophet myself. These people came to me as they wanted to experience the gift of prophecy and learn how to evangelize by using their new prophetic gift. Everyone I prayed for has received this wonderful gift. It makes me wonder if my prayer called up the gift of prophecy in their lives. Or did the process of just coming to me and saying a prayer stir up their faith so that they realized the gift that was **already** in them? I personally believe that every Christian is equipped to minister in the prophetic, for Scripture says that we are created to do good works.

Hebrews 13:21 . . . make you complete in every good work to do His will, working in you what is well pleasing in His sight, through Jesus Christ, to whom be glory forever and ever. Amen.

Many people are preaching, holding conferences, and writing books about how one can be ready for this new anointing and power. Christians move from one conference to another, thinking that this is what reinforces their divine gift. Sadly, there seems to be a thriving market to endow believers with everything that they already have.

Colossians 2:8-10 - Beware lest anyone cheat you through philosophy and empty deceit, according to the tradition of men, according to the basic principles of the world, and not according to Christ. For in Him dwells all the fullness of the Godhead bodily; and you are complete in Him, who is the head of all principality and power.

Many of us think that we need to be like another famous person. Many of us think that if we could only have Heidi Baker, Rick Joyner, or Kris Vallotton pray for us, then we might walk in a more powerful anointing, do more good, and sin a whole lot less. However, Scripture says that we are already perfect, complete, and faultless from the day we were born again and filled with the Holy Spirit.

Jude 1:24 - Now to Him who is able to keep you from stumbling, and to present you faultless before the presence of His glory with exceeding joy . . . .

It might be one thing for me to string together a whole lot of verses, saying that you are perfect and already complete. Even so, when you lack the power to cast out demons, when you cannot pray for someone to receive healing, and when you are still caught in sin, the circumstances tend to argue with the assertion that you are perfect and complete.

But does that really hold weight? Just because these conditions are saying that you are a sinner and not powerful, does that mean that you are weak and unfit for the Kingdom?

Evangelists teach people how to share the Gospel with their friends and family. Effective healers teach others how to move in healing like they do. Teachers of the Word teach and equip the saints. The fivefold ministry of apostles, prophets, evangelists, pastors, and teachers equips the body and prepares them for the works of ministry.

I have written a book called *The Parables of Jesus Made Simple: Updated and Expanded Edition*. In that book, I teach the reader how to obey the parables of Jesus and live them out today.

I have also written a book on how to deliver a prophecy and how to find out if you are called to be a prophet. *The Prophetic Supernatural Experience* has equipped a lot of people to move in the life of the prophetic.

Wisdom can be taught. People can be perfected in life by simply learning that they are already perfect because of Christ.

Colossians 1:28 . . . Him we preach, warning every man and teaching every man in all wisdom, that we may present every man perfect in Christ Jesus

Some people reading this might say, "No matter how many verses you quote, my experience in my Christian life bears out the fact that I am neither perfect nor complete." Not knowing the truth of who you are might be the very reason that you and I are not walking in the path of perfection and completeness.

James says that when we are experienced in being patient, we become perfect and complete, and we have everything that we need to do a great job for God in the world.

James 1:4 - But let patience have its perfect work, that you may be perfect and complete, lacking nothing.

The Christian life can be somewhat of a maze. Sometimes, we seem to be running around in circles, lost and wondering which way we should go. I once asked an experienced apostle, a man who would not openly confess that he was an apostle. "Why can't there be a book on how to live the perfect Christian life?" He said that if such a book were written, the devil would have counterfeited it, and the counterfeit would be the bestseller. I was upset but understood that we all need the Holy Spirit to lead us into truth.

Living the Christian life as well as embodying Christianity is not always a walk in the park, for the path might be filled with danger and suffering.

Jesus knew that his disciples would go through these hardships, and he warned them beforehand. Through suffering and trials, we learn patience and develop character. We mature and eventually seek peace. The more we understand these Scriptures and truths, the stronger and more effective we become.

1 Peter 5:10 - But may the God of all grace, who called us to His eternal glory by Christ Jesus, after you have suffered a while, perfect, establish, strengthen, and settle you.

It is possible to be perfect and complete. If it were not possible, it would mean that the Scriptures we have looked up to would not be in the Bible. When we look at our own lives, at our struggles, our sins, and our lack of power, we assume that we are not complete. But if you think about it, if the same Holy Spirit that resided in Christ resides in us, then it is possible that we can be complete and perfect as well.

2 Corinthians 13:11 - Finally, brethren, farewell. Become complete. Be of good comfort, be of one mind, live in peace; and the God of love and peace will be with you.

If you knew Joseph Prince, Joyce Meyer, or Heidi Baker personally, and you showed them this chapter and asked them if it is theologically correct that we can really be complete and perfect, you might be pleasantly surprised at their response.

One entity in the world does not want you to know these things, and many people in the world might preach something different, especially if they are selling a book to you. But wouldn't it be cool to meditate on these verses, accept them, and start to move into the place where we live in the truth and not walk in the error that Satan would have us believe? I am the first person to admit that I am not walking in this truth like I should.

Colossians 4:12 - Epaphras, who is one of you, a bondservant of Christ, greets you, always laboring fervently for you in prayers, that you may stand perfect and complete in all the will of God.

Chapter 7 – You Are Holy and Blameless

In the last chapter, you learned that we are already perfect and complete. Many people, despite the Scriptures shown, might disagree but not because it isn't possible or isn't right. The reason that people disagree is that for some reason, I have not heard this subject preached very often. The idea that we do not have to buy that book or to attend that conference and the thought that we do not have to have that person with a great and powerful anointing lay hands on us seems foreign to us.

In my own life, no one prayed for me to receive the gift of prophecy. I just started to prophesy. No one anointed me to be a prophet, and no mentor coached me in the office of prophet. I struggled, learned, listened to Jesus and the Holy Spirit, and finally matured, and was promoted by God into the office. No church appointed me, taught me, or ordained me. I was called, trained, equipped, and ordained by Jesus Christ, the Anointed One.

This same Spirit that anointed Jesus is effective in making us holy. The Holy Spirit does a great work in us when we accept Jesus Christ as our personal Saviour.

Once again, your mind might argue with the idea; your reasoning and the storehouse of your experience and past teachings might scream bloody murder, but Scripture declares that you are now holy.

Colossians 1:21-23 - And you, who once were alienated and enemies in your mind by wicked works, yet now He has reconciled in the body of His flesh through death, to present you holy, and blameless, and above reproach in His sight—if indeed you continue in the faith, grounded and steadfast, and are not moved away from the hope of the gospel which you heard, which was preached to every creature under Heaven, of which I, Paul, became a minister.

I am not sure about you, but as I write this, my own mind is screaming, "But what about that sin you committed last week?" My own unrenewed mind that does not accept the truth of the Scriptures wants to tell me that this is a pile of garbage.

My mind, screaming that I am not holy, is the same as the butterfly's mind screaming and saying that he is not a butterfly but still a caterpillar. However, Scripture declares that as we share in Jesus' death and resurrection, we have become a new creation. As a new creation, our old, sinful nature has been crucified with Christ, and we have arisen as holy.

Colossians 3:12 - Therefore, as the elect of God, holy and beloved, put on tender mercies, kindness, humility, meekness, long suffering;

Many people are saved through the grace of Christ and are far from kind, humble, meek, and long-suffering. Many people in the Christian faith seem to lack many of the fruit of the Spirit, so how can we call them holy? The fact is that, while we can miss it, when it comes to refined character, the Holy Spirit that inhabits our spirits misses nothing.

As Christians, we are called to be holy and set apart. We should no longer be taken in by the lusts of the world. As a new creation, we should develop in the fruit of the Spirit. We should start to obey the teachings of Jesus and choose willingly to live in love toward God and our fellow man. When we are perfected in love, when everything we do is motivated by love, then we act out what is ours at our new birth—holiness.

1 Peter 1:15-16 - But as He who called you is holy, you also be holy in all your conduct, because it is written, “Be holy, for I am holy.”

Would Peter tell his followers and the readers of his epistles to be holy if it were not possible? Would God in the Old Testament that Peter quotes above ask his people to be holy if it were not possible? Once again, our mind wants to argue. Our actions, the sin in our lives, and our former teachings scream at us and say that being holy is just not possible in this world. But I do not think that Peter would ask us to be holy if he himself were not holy.

If we cannot be made whole and achieve holiness in this world by the enabling of the Holy Spirit, why would God want us to be so? Many people are happier not knowing the truth. They know that they are sinful and live a life of failure. But at the same time, they cannot accept that there is any way out of it. We live lives of quiet desperation, wearing faces of suffering and wondering like Paul did, who can deliver us from this body of sin (Romans 7)?

Before the earth was created, God desired that he might have holy people set apart in love for him and for others.

Ephesians 1:4 - Just as He chose us in Him before the foundation of the world, that we should be holy and without blame before Him in love.

Is it too hard to accept that the Holy Spirit gives us the power to walk in perfection? Scripture says that every person has the choice to sin or not to sin. We all are given a way out of our sin, a way of escape. Paul has encouraged all of us to pursue holiness.

Hebrews 12:14 - Pursue peace with all people, and holiness, without which no one will see the Lord.

If both Peter and Paul compelled us to be holy, and they knew what they were talking about, then do you think that we might have missed this message? Holiness is not only possible, but we can make it a discipline in our Christian lives.

Many people will use the above Scripture to beat Christians over the head and warn them that they will not enter heaven without living holy lives. This Scripture, if you have heard it, might not be one of your favorite ones and might make you fear for your eternal salvation. That is not why the Scripture was written. It was given to encourage us to pursue holiness and to tell us that it is possible to be holy.

As believers, we host the very presence of God. As one who is saved, we have the Holy Spirit living in us, and therefore, we are his temple. God calls our temple holy, so why don't we all act that way?

Chapter 8 – You Are Inhabitants of a Brand New Kingdom

Many people, even after they are saved or born again still continue to live by the rules of the kingdom of this world. They are unaware that they are in a new kingdom, that the rules have changed, and that they do not have to perform the same way anymore.

Colossians 1:13-14 - He has delivered us from the power of darkness and conveyed us into the kingdom of the Son of His love, in whom we have redemption through His blood, the forgiveness of sins.

Instead of being a sinner, they are now a saint and a citizen of heaven. Instead of being filthy, they are washed clean as wool, as white as snow, and are righteous and holy. Instead of being alone, they are the elect and chosen of God. Instead of being worthless based on their job or education, they are special, chosen, and holy.

The new kingdom operates in a new way. There is little need to strive to be loved. You are loved without measure. You are the beloved of God, and you are a righteous son or daughter. You are a precious son or daughter of God, and no more do you have to perform to be holy and set apart. What Christ did set you apart and made you special. Even if you are currently struggling with addictions, your identity is based on what Christ says about you and not on what you do.

Instead of coming to God with special duties and sacrifices, you can rest in the fact that Christ, who is sinless and perfect, laid down his life and made a sacrifice for you that was forever accepted in your place.

Instead of having no power or ability to fight the wrong things that we are tempted with each day, we are given the Holy Spirit to enable us to walk in perfection and holiness. Where once we were bound and held by sin and bondages, Christ's power came to break every chain and set the captives free.

The enemy wants you ignorant of this new reality. He would prefer that you think that while you sin, you are a sinner. He does not want you to know that you now belong to the Kingdom of Light and that you now have a new nature that does not need to fall into sin. As long as you are convinced that you are a sinner and not a righteous saint, you will sadly remain in a sinful lifestyle.

Many people teach that a person who has been born into the Kingdom of God can lose their salvation if they sin, and therefore, they can go to hell. Quite a number of very popular preachers say that a person can be born into the Kingdom of God and then fall away and go back into the kingdom of darkness. This is a sad teaching that puts fear into people. This fear, rather than releasing people into righteous living, keeps them bound in a sinful lifestyle.

If you continue to say that you are a sinner, you will continue to sin. If you instead say that you are righteous and holy, soon enough, your body and mind will be transformed and begin to line up with the new confession, even if you still struggle to believe this new confession.

Chapter 9 – You Are Righteous, Peaceful, and Joyful

Many people think that their pastor or priest is righteous, but they do not see themselves as particularly righteous. They assume that because they have sin in their life, they are not righteous. They assume that only people who do not commit any wrong can be righteous. With that in mind, many Christians live quiet lives of desperation, wondering what is different about them and wondering why they were not saved from sin.

2 Corinthians 5:21 - For He made Him who knew no sin to be sin for us, that we might become the righteousness of God in Him.

The truth is that we have been made righteous through the death and resurrection of Jesus Christ. God made Jesus sin so that we might have a divine exchange and wear his robe of righteousness. Once again, preachers and Satan want us to believe that if we are sinning, then we are not righteous. People are left so confused, but this verse tells us as plain as day that Jesus became sin so that we might be made righteous.

What is the point of the empowering of the Holy Spirit if one cannot defeat sin? The way to defeat sin is not to strive against it but to see yourself as righteous and live from that mindset. When you understand that you are perfect, complete, holy, chosen, set apart, and righteous, your mind begins to grab a hold of the fact that it is possible to be a new creation and to walk like it.

Years ago, no man had ever run the mile in under four minutes. It was assumed impossible for a man to do. One day, Roger Banister ran a mile in under four minutes. What the world of runners thought was impossible suddenly became possible. Since then, hundreds of people have run the mile in under four minutes. People only needed to believe that it was possible. People need to know that it is possible to live a life free of sin.

I have met two men who confessed to me that they rarely sinned. I was shocked to find that sin was a very rare occurrence for them. Rather than making me depressed, I became excited. I knew if they could do it, it was possible for me as well.

We discussed that Paul and Peter urged people to be holy. We agreed that Paul and Peter would not be asking people to do something that they were not already doing. Don't you see? When you know you are seen as righteous by God, you can more easily conform into that image.

We are not meant to go through our lives living in shame, guilt, and condemnation. We are instead meant to live in joy and peace through the manifest presence of Jesus resting in our lives.

Romans 14:17 - For the kingdom of God is not eating and drinking, but righteousness and peace and joy in the Holy Spirit.

Many people are crippled with guilt and shame. Since I was addicted to pornography for thirty-six years, I lived in a constant cycle of shame, guilt, and condemnation. Every few days, I fell again and ran away from God and his presence for a day or two. I finally learned that I was forgiven and loved despite my sin. I then reached the point where I could walk in the Spirit and overcome the addiction.

People should know us for the joy that is within us. People should see us as happy and joyful. People should know that the Christian life has real rewards and is a life of peace in the midst of the same storms that batter the lives of those who are not saved. People who are not saved should look at us and see something that they want. They should not see us as the angry, upset, religious, and judgmental people that many of them see.

It is possible to walk in the knowledge that you are loved, accepted, and righteous even in the midst of sinning. I needed to come to a point where I knew that I was loved no matter what I was doing, to finally reach a point where I could allow God to give me the grace to overcome my addictions. As you read this, are you fully convinced that you are loved by Jesus and his Father? My prayer is that you will grasp the depth of this truth.

2017 UPDATE - When I wrote this book a couple of years ago, I had experienced a measure of freedom, but I fell back into porn after about six months of freedom.

Being set free was a miracle, but this miracle was birthed in the knowledge and understanding that I was considered a righteous son **before** I was actually set free.

Jesus told a parable about a feast in Matthew 22:1-14. At the feast, people were given wedding clothes, and they were seated. Each of the guests was given the same robe so that every person, no matter their wealth or social standing, was dressed the same. However, a man was found who did not have on the wedding clothes. Although he was given the clothes, he decided not to put them on and dress like the other people. The host of the feast had him kicked out.

This man represents a person who has been given the robes of the righteousness of Christ yet has decided to live in his own self-righteous acts and deeds. Jesus wants you to accept that you are seen by him as righteous, and he wants you to work that out in your life until you have overcome and really are living a life free from sin.

Preachers preach all about the Ten Commandments and the law of God and say that you have to stop doing certain things to be righteous. However, you cannot ever be motivated not to do something by being told you cannot do it. People who preach the law instead of teaching you how to walk in love and righteousness actually strengthen the hold of sin in your life.

You are free to be righteous, joyful, and peaceful. Do you want to be?

Chapter 10 – Coming to True Repentance

I'm pleased that we've covered the content regarding identity in the last four chapters and laid some ground work for who you are and for how God sees you. Until you can accept who you really are in God's eyes, you will struggle to break free of prostitution and pornography.

I shared briefly that you have to come to a place of true repentance. You can't just say that you're sorry, cry crocodile tears, and promise, "I won't do it again. Jesus, I feel so bad. I am so sorry." It's not acceptable to just feel sorry for yourself and hope that it all stops. I had to reach a point where I addressed the prostitution. I had to reach a point where I realized that I was sinning against the girls. I was sinning against myself, against God's finances, against the temple of the Lord, and against God.

You might need some help to feel convicted about your pornography addiction. You might need to read a book by a porn star who's come out of the industry and become a Christian and who has been set free of the related shame and guilt.

Perhaps you need to get involved and support sex trafficking organizations since sex trafficking uses girls for pornography and prostitution. Perhaps you need to read the stories of women who are abused and raped. You might need to hear the real stories of shame and degradation and how terrible their lives were in order to find the motivation to be free.

The more you can empathize with the women who are used in pornography, the more you can understand that it isn’t a glamorous life. The more you can get to the truth of the matter, the better off you'll be and the better position that you'll be in so that you're truly sorry for the women who are being abused and trafficked to make porn. You will be truly sorry for the prostitute that you are using. Unless you can reach a point where you understand that you're abusing prostitutes by seeing them and that you're not really a nice person, you might not get free. Your money isn’t really worth what you're doing to the girl, and you're abusing, hurting, and taking advantage of them. You must understand that you're really sinning, and you're upsetting God, and she wasn’t made for you to have sex with outside of marriage.

If you're a married man, you have to understand that four people are involved.

- Your wife is involved, and you're committing adultery.
- The woman that you're sleeping with is involved because you're committing adultery with her and raping her.
- As the temple of the Holy Spirit, you and your finances are involved.
- God is involved, and his heart is broken by how you are treating his daughter and treating yourself.

If you're sleeping with prostitutes and you're married, you're in one holy mess. If you're viewing pornography and you're married, you're upsetting your wife and destroying the intimacy of your marriage. You're defiling the marriage bed, and you're committing spiritual and sexual adultery against your wife. You're abusing your own flesh, and you're displeasing God. God loves you, and you are his child, and he adores you. But he doesn't like you to hurt yourself. He doesn't like you going against his commandments. He's a holy God, and he wants you to live a holy life.

You need to weigh and consider all those things to reach a place with God where you can say, "I really want to walk away from this." If you're addicted to prostitutes, perhaps you can pray a prayer in church and publicly confess without spelling out what your sin is. You can say a prayer out loud or in a group among witnesses and pray that you are set free of what's troubling you. I also encourage you to share with friends about this issue. Find supportive people who can pray with you and cover you. But you have to reach a stage where you're at the end of yourself, where you can admit to yourself that you cannot do it alone. You must come to grips with the fact that you need a sovereign act of God to help you.

I thought that I could solve the prostitution problem by finding other things to spend my money on so that I didn't have enough money to spend on prostitutes. That only worked for a while until Satan hit me with strong temptation. As soon as I was paid, I was off to see a prostitute again. It worked for a few weeks but that kind of "self-control" doesn't work in a long run.

You have to reach a stage where you're at the end of yourself. You have to say, "As for me and my house, I want to serve the Lord. I want to walk away from iniquity. Lord, please help me."

Chapter 11 – God's Grace Is the Answer

Remember Ephesians 2:8-9 that says, "For by grace we've been saved through faith, that not of yourselves, it's a gift of God. Not by works, lest anyone should boast." For by grace through faith, we've been saved from pornography or an addiction to prostitutes.

So what saved you? The power and the grace and the enabling of Jesus Christ. How do you access it? Through faith. And how do you do it? You don't do it through your own efforts or striving or your own decision not to view pornography and not to have the computer on when your wife is out. You don't do it by denying yourself of money so that you don't have money to see prostitutes.

You're saved by God's enabling power through grace; you access it through faith, and you don't do it through yourself or your own clever works or ideas, such as denying yourself of certain things.

You **don't** do it by yourself.

You **can't** do it by yourself.

You have to come to the end of yourself where you accept and say to Jesus, in true repentance, "I can't do this. I want to do this, but I need your grace. I need you to help take away the temptation from me. I need you to work through your angels and deliver me through grace so that I can walk free of this."

You don't do it through works. You don't achieve it through works. I didn't achieve it through putting pornography filters on my computer. I could never get them to work. If you can get filtering software for pornography on your home computers and on your work computer, by all means, do that. However, if you find that this doesn't work for you, you need to repent and come before God and cast yourself on his mercy seat. Cast yourself on his grace and say that through faith, you want to be set free. Through his faith, through his grace, and through his love for you, God will act. It won't be something that you can boast about in and of yourself.

I want to make it clear that this is nothing that I did. When I repented of prostitution years ago, I just said a simple prayer. Formerly, when I was paid, I was tempted ten out of ten or at least eight out of ten. After I prayed that prayer, the next time I was paid, the temptation dropped to two out of ten. I wasn't even tempted, and it didn't seem that powerful. Before then, a big demon was on my back that used to pull me down to sin. I was powerless against this demonic force. When I properly repented of the temptation, that demon left. Whatever was causing the temptation to be eight out of ten and even stronger finally left me.

Pornography was the same. I was finally set free by God when I came to the end of myself and trusted God and his grace and accepted myself and walked free from the sin. I had to daily accept that God loved me and that I'm perfect and righteous.

Until I accepted who I was in Christ, I wasn't able to get free. When I accepted that I was perfect, holy, and blameless, when I accepted that I was in a new kingdom and that I didn't have to sin, God gave me the grace to walk in his new kingdom.

You have to understand that you're saved through grace with access by faith. You have to understand that you're not saved by works, so you can’t boast about it. I'm the last person who can boast. I had a thirty-six-year addiction to pornography, and I didn’t do anything to overcome it. I repented and came to the end of myself. I learned who I was in Christ; this was one of the keys. If you’re sick of hearing me say that I had to come to the end of myself, you have to be that sick of yourself to get rid of this sin.

I encourage you to read *Your Identity in Christ*, the book from which some of this material came. Learn who you are and what is possible in your life. Start to move into that identity and come to a place where you truly repent. Come to a place where you're at the end of yourself and then cast yourself onto the grace of God and ask him to deliver you. I went through that process. It was hard and took many years of suffering and trials, but the beautiful thing is that all things work together for good for those who love God and who are called according to his purpose as it says in Romans 8:28. The beautiful thing is that God can use my life to encourage you, to show you through my transparency and my honesty that I really struggled, that I really cried, and that I went through many years of challenges.

Ephesians 2:10 says, "For we are His workmanship, created in Christ Jesus for good works, which God prepared beforehand that we should work in them." Part of my good work is writing and producing books, including spending a couple of thousand dollars of my own money to publish this book to encourage you to walk free as well.

Chapter 12 – Walking out Your Freedom

If you have occasions where you are free from pornography for a month or even for three months, if you repent and find the grace to walk in freedom, the temptation might seem to leave or diminish for a little while. You might be free for a few months, but then you sin again and fall back into the same struggles. Dust yourself off, brush yourself off, and don't restart the clock at day one. Say that you've been free for three months with one fall. Keep counting the months until you're free for a much longer stretch of time. This is important because it helps you reframe your thinking and empowers you to continue to overcome.

I have found when that when I had a length of time that I was free from pornography, I could not boast about my victory or share about it with everyone. The enemy likes to come in to take away your victory and come against people who are prideful. If you start to boast and share that you are finally free from pornography, you might sadly go back into it. I suggest that you keep your freedom private and just walk it out for a season. I was free for a few months from pornography, and I thought I was totally free. I then shared it with my whole church, and I fell back into it.

Take one day and one step at a time. After you are free, if you fall back into it, don't condemn yourself or wallow in guilt and shame. Instead, go back and meditate on the fact that you're righteous, holy, blameless, and joyful. Start to identify with who you really are and who the Bible says you are as a son of God, as a righteous son, as a holy son of the Father. Continue to explore your identity.

If you fall, you might need more inner healing to clean up some more problem areas that might be causing you to slip back into addiction. One thing is for sure. If you have struggled with an addiction for any amount of time, whether it be pornography or prostitutes, Satan doesn't want you free, and he will use anything or try anything to get you back into it.

I received a prophecy that told me that I was free and that Satan realized that he had lost his battle with me. However, he now wanted to play a long game with me. He would be patient and wait to ensnare me again or come against me in a surprise attack. I needed to be vigilant and wary with a heavy guard up at all times because Satan prowls around like a hungry lion.

Take one step at a time. If you have people you have shared your struggles with, you can share with them that you've been free of pornography for a week and then two weeks, three weeks, a month, two months, three months, four months, six months. Share your victories and your freedom with them.

Some of those people might be struggling with the same sin, so they will be encouraged when they hear that someone else has overcome the same issue. Since I gained freedom but then fell, I was waiting on the Holy Spirit for the right time and inspiration to write this book.

Earlier this morning, I sat down and wrote the chapter titles for this book. The Lord then led me to my book, *Your Identity in Christ*, and I initially reviewed the book just to find some Scripture references so that I could dictate this book. As I read some of the passages, the Holy Spirit showed me, "No, just cut and paste four chapters from that book into this book and have that as the foundation for this book. People can learn from that and encourage them to go and read the whole book for themselves."

Don't beat yourself up if you fall into sin. Instead of counting your days of freedom from your slip up, count them from the beginning. Don't say that you've been free for three months, but now you've only been free for a day. Say that you've been free for three months and you've had one slip up. See if you can stay free for another three months and then say that you've been free for six months with one fall rather than three months-three months. You can see if that works for you.

I pray that this book has really encouraged you. Like I said, I struggled for thirty-six years with pornography and twenty-five years with prostitution. I'm far from a perfect man. If you read any more of my books, you will realize that I'm always transparent and honest.

A friend of mine, Michael Van Vlymen, said that what he really loves about me is that I'm willing to throw myself under a bus to make a point. This is very true. I love you all.

I have invested a couple of thousand dollars into producing this book to give you hope. You need to know that you're loved. I spent this money to encourage you that, one day, you can be free, too.

To sum everything up, here is what led to my freedom:

- Inner healing
- Deliverance
- Proper theology
- True repentance and
- The grace of God.

I pray that these lead you to freedom as well.

I'd love to hear from you

One of the ways that you can bless me as a writer is by writing an honest and candid review of my book on Amazon. I always read the reviews of my books, and I would love to hear what you have to say about this one.

Before I buy a book, I read the reviews first. You can make an informed decision about a book when you have read enough honest reviews from readers. One way to help me sell this book and to give me positive feedback is by writing a review for me. It doesn't cost you a thing but helps me and the future readers of this book enormously.

If you would like to sow money into my book-writing ministry and would like to sow a portion into a book, please visit my website and ask me what projects I am working on.

Visit my website at http://personal-prophecy-today.com to read my blog, request a life-coaching session, request your own personal prophecy, request a visit to heaven, or to receive a personal message from your angel. All of the funds raised through my ministry website will go toward the books that I write and self-publish. Feel free to sow money into my book-publishing ministry as the Holy Spirit leads you.

Please feel free to contact me at my personal email address at survivors.sanctuary@gmail.com to write to me about this book or to share any other thoughts.

You can also friend request me on Facebook at Matthew Robert Payne. Please send me a message if we have no friends in common as a lot of scammers now send me friend requests.

You can also do me a huge favor and share this book on Facebook as a recommended book to read. This will help me and other readers.

How to Sponsor a Book Project

If you have been blessed by this book, you might consider sponsoring a book for me. It normally costs me between fifteen hundred and two thousand dollars or more to produce each book that I write, depending on the length of the book.

If you seek the Holy Spirit about financing a book for me, I know that the Lord would be eternally grateful to you. Consider how much this book has blessed you and then think of hundreds or even thousands of people who would be blessed by a book of mine. As you are probably aware, the vast majority of my books are ninety-nine cents on Kindle, which proves to you that book writing is indeed a ministry for me and not a money- making venture. I would be very happy if you supported me in this.

If you have any questions for me or if you want to know what projects I am currently working on that your money might finance, you can write to me at **survivors.sanctuary@gmail.com** and ask me for more information. I would be pleased to give you more details about my projects. You can sow any amount to my ministry by simply sending me money via the PayPal link at this address: http://personal-prophecy-today.com/support-my-ministry/ You can be sure that your support, no matter the amount, will be used for the publishing of helpful Christian books for people to read.

Other Books by Matthew Robert Payne

The Prophetic Supernatural Experience

Prophetic Evangelism Made Simple

Your Identity in Christ

His Redeeming Love- A Memoir

Writing and Self-Publishing Christian Nonfiction

Coping with your Pain and Suffering

Living for Eternity

Jesus Speaking Today

Great Cloud of Witnesses Speak

My Radical Encounters with Angels

Finding Intimacy with Jesus Made Simple

My Radical Encounters with Angels- Book Two

A Beginner's Guide to the Prophetic

Michael Jackson Speaks from Heaven

7 Keys to Intimacy with Jesus

Conversations with God: Book 1

Optimistic Visions of Revelation

Conversations with God: Book 2

Finding Your Purpose in Christ

Influencing your World for Christ: Practical Everyday Evangelism

Deep Calls unto Deep: Answering Questions on the Prophetic

My Visits to the Galactic Council of Heaven

The Parables of Jesus Made Simple: Updated and Expanded Edition

Great Cloud of Witnesses Speak: Old and New

Walking under an Open Heaven

A Message from My Angel

Interviews with the Two Witnesses: Enoch and Elijah Speak

You can find my published books on my

Amazon author page here:
http://tinyurl.com/jq3h893

Upcoming Books

Mary Magdalene Speaks from Heaven: A Divine Revelation

About Matthew Robert Payne

Matthew was raised in a Baptist church and was led to the Lord at the tender age of eight. He has experienced some pain and darkness in his life, which has given him a deep compassion and love for all people.

Today, he runs a Facebook group called "Open Heavens and Intimacy with Jesus." Matthew has a commission from the Lord to train up prophets and to mentor others in the Christian faith. He does this through his Facebook posts and by writing relevant books on the Christian faith.

God has commissioned him to write at least fifty books in his life, and he spends his days writing and earning the money to self-publish. You can support him by donating money at http://personal-prophecy-today.com or by requesting any of his other services available through his ministry website.

It is Matthew's prayer that this book has blessed you, and he hopes it will lead you into a deeper and more intimate relationship with God.

www.ingramcontent.com/pod-product-compliance
Ingram Content Group UK Ltd.
Pitfield, Milton Keynes, MK11 3LW, UK
UKHW020138250726
13967UKWH00002B/733

9 781684 114030